Organic

Antibiotics and Antivirals

Recipes for Healing

Disclaimer and Terms of Use:

Effort has been made to ensure that the information in this book is accurate and complete, however, the author and the publisher do not warrant the accuracy of the information, text and graphics contained within the book due to the rapidly changing nature of science, research, known and unknown facts and internet. The Author and the publisher do not hold any responsibility for errors, omissions or contrary interpretation of the subject matter herein. This book is presented solely for motivational and informational purposes only.

Contents

Introduction

Thank you for downloading this book, *"Healing Naturally: 25 Organic Antibiotics and Antivirals Recipes for healing"*.

This book is all about taking care of your health and treating infections the natural way. The body is always at risk for infections. Viruses and bacteria abound in the environment, which can cause illnesses at any time. The immediate answer for most of these illnesses is pharmaceutical antiviral and antibacterial drugs. These chemical treatments are effective, but its use also poses a few dangers. These drugs cause side effects ranging from minor discomforts to serious, potential life-threatening conditions.

Prolific use of antibiotics to treat common cough, flu, colds and sore throat can also cause the development of superbugs. These are microorganisms that have developed resistance to antibiotics. Superbugs cause very serious infections that are near impossible to treat and can be life-threatening.

In order to avoid these scenarios, turn to nature. There are many foods that have natural antibiotic and antiviral effects that can effectively cure infections, without the side effects.

Read this book and find out what foods can be taken to fight infections the natural way. Also, you get a few recipes on how to use these foods to cure those infections.

Read on and learn.

Again, thank you for downloading.

Chapter 1 Natural Antibiotic Foods & General Recipes

Antibacterial and antiviral foods contain compounds that have natural abilities to kill bacteria, fungus and viruses that cause illnesses. They also stimulate the body's immune system to increase the body's ability to fight against infections and recover from sickness.

Honey

Honey was the first antimicrobial food ever used to treat infections; long before the first antimicrobial drugs were invented. Raw honey has very potent antibacterial and antiviral properties. Research has shown that honey contains several compounds working together to combat infections such as defensin-1 (antimicrobial peptide), methylglyoxal, and hydrogen peroxide. It also has high sugar concentrations and low pH.

Another study found that honey stimulates the natural release of hydrogen peroxide in the body, which kills pathogens. Experts are also considering the use of honey to combat infections caused by antibiotic-resistant microorganisms.

Horseradish

This root vegetable has a very strong, spicy taste that goes well with different kinds of foods. Besides culinary uses, horseradish has very potent antimicrobial properties. One of which is that it can be used to treat different kinds of respiratory and urinary tract infections.

Lemon

This citrus fruit has long been known to have antibacterial properties. The compounds tetrazine and coumarin in lemons are effective against certain pathogens, making it effective against both internal and external infections.

Pineapple

Pineapples are full of compounds that have very potent antibacterial properties. The compound bromelain is effective at treating throat and mouth infections. There have also been documented cases wherein pineapples were used as a part of the treatment of diphtheria in the 1950s.

Milk curd

Milk curd is very effective at fighting off bacterial infections. The fermentation process used to create milk curds also produces beneficial bacteria that can help fight infections in the body. These probiotic bacteria also help in restoring the balance of the normal intestinal bacterial flora.

Turmeric

The health benefits of turmeric have a strong scientific data to back it up. Studies have shown that turmeric is effective against specific pathogens like *Bacillus cereus, Bacillus subtilis, Bacillus coagulans, Escherichia coli, Pseudomonas aeroginosa and Staphylococcus aureus.*

Ginger

This root has long been used as a treatment against bacteria that cause respiratory infections. Research found that the compounds called gingerols are effective in eliminating several gram-negative bacteria from the body.

Onion

This pungent root bulb contains potent antibacterial sulfur compounds. These compounds are effective at fighting several pathogens, most particularly *Staphylococcus aureus*. Onions can be used externally and internally to treat several kinds of infections. It can either be ingested or applied topically on infected areas.

Garlic

This is considered as one of the most potent antimicrobial foods. It contains sulfur compounds that are effective in fighting several infections. These compounds can kill bacteria, as well as worms, yeast and fungi. It can also fight Candida overgrowth (yeast infection).

Coconut oil

The medium chain fatty acid found in coconut oil, called lauric acid, has been found to have potent antimicrobial properties.

Cabbage

Cabbages contain compounds that can effectively kill infectious bacteria, and they are most effective against urinary tract infections. Studies have also found that cabbage juice is effective in controlling bacterial populations of *H. pylori*, the main cause of stomach ulcers.

Herbs

Herbs also contain compounds that are effective in fighting off bacterial, fungal and viral infections. Here are some of the herbs that have antibacterial properties:

- Thyme
- Rosemary
- Mint leaves
- Cinnamon
- Basil
- Sage
- Chervil
- Oregano

- Lemon balm

- Cumin

- Cloves

- Tarragon

- Bay leaf

- Caraway seed

- Chili peppers

- Dill

- Marjoram

- Coriander

- Nutmeg

- Pepper

- Cardamom

Manuka Honey

This type of honey is obtained from the nectar of the flower of the Manuka bush, a wild plant that is native only to New Zealand. Manuka honey has very effective antibacterial properties. It is known to stimulate a chemical reaction within the body which induces the natural production of hydrogen peroxide, an effective antiseptic that kills pathogens.

Uses of Manuka honey:

- Apply the honey directly on wounds to discourage bacterial infection and promote faster healing.

- To treat acne, use Manuka honey as a face mask. Leave it on for 15 to 30 minutes before rinsing well with water.

- For seasonal allergies, gastritis, stomach ulcers and infections, add a tablespoon of Manuka honey to your tea or food.

- For cough, sinusitis, and sore throats, a tablespoon of Manuka honey 3 times daily will help alleviate the symptoms.

Apple Cider Vinegar

Apple cider vinegar (also called ACV or cider vinegar) is made from crushed apples. The resulting juice is fermented into vinegar by adding cultured yeast and bacteria.

During the second fermentation process, bacteria that form acetic acid are added. All the added bacteria during the fermentation process are responsible for the healing benefits of apple cider vinegar. The color of ACV ranges from pale to medium amber, depending on how long it is fermented for.

Uses of Apple Cider Vinegar:

- As an antiseptic for treating acne and other similar skin problems. To use ACV, dilute it with equal amounts of water and apply on the face. Allow it to sit on the skin for 5 minutes before rinsing.

- For dandruff (fungal infection of the scalp caused by *Malassezia furfur* fungus), dilute with equal amounts of water and massage on the scalp.

- For yeast infections in women, add 2 tablespoons to a small basin of water and use as a douche. Use this with caution as it can irritate the vaginal mucosa and disrupt the normal vaginal bacterial flora.

Oregano Oil Uses

Oregano oil, as the name implies, comes from the oregano. The oil is extracted from the oregano leaves through steam distillation. There are actually 40 different species of oregano herbs known to exist, but among them, the oil from Oreganum Vulgare is considered as the most potent.

The antibacterial properties of oregano can be used in the following ways:

1. Relieve swollen glands and sore throat by diluting equal parts oregano oil and water. Apply topically over the throat.

2. Mix 4 drops of oregano oil and 1 drop clover oil (or just use 5 drops of oregano oil) and put them in a capsule. Take a capsule 3 times each day until symptoms of flu and cold disappear.

3. Place 15 drops of oregano oil in a capsule. Take 1 capsule three times a day to protect against bronchitis and strep throat infections.

4. Place 5 drops of oregano oil in a capsule. Take 3 times a day to effectively and quickly treat urinary tract infections.

5. Take oregano oil internally to fight off chronic fungal infections.

6. Prepare 1/8 cup of water and add 1 drop of oregano oil. Gargle then swallow to relieve sore throat.

7. Rub a diluted mixture of oregano and thyme oil over aching muscles caused by viral infections.

8. Mix 1 part oregano oil and 5 parts olive oil. Place in a dropper bottle. For the first few hours of flu, place 3 drops under the tongue every 15 minutes. Then place 3 drops under the tongue once every hour for the next 24 hours. Then take several times a day for the next few days until full recovery from a flu infection.

9. Dilute oregano oil to 50% with a carrier oil. Apply on the skin surface affected with athlete's foot and other skin fungal infections. Use twice a day, every day.

10. Place diluted oregano oil in a diffuser. Spray in the room to clear the air of infective microorganisms.

Chapter 2 Natural Antibiotics Recipes for Sore Throat

Sore throat is a condition wherein the throat becomes painful, irritated, and at times, swollen. It may be due to an infection. It may also be a consequence of frequent coughing.

Foods that relieve sore throat

Apple cider vinegar

This is an effective remedy against viral and bacterial infections. It creates an acidic environment inside the body, which is inhospitable to bacteria and viruses. It also has anti-inflammatory properties, which can reduce the swelling in the throat.

Raw honey or Manuka honey

Honey has potent antiviral, antifungal, and antibacterial properties, effective against pathogens that cause sore throat. Honey also coats the mucosal lining of the throat, which provides relief and protection from further irritation.

Lemon

Lemon has astringent properties that help treat sore throat. The compounds shrink the swelling of the throat tissues. It also creates an acidic environment hostile to bacteria and viruses.

Wheatgrass juice

This liquid is rich in chlorophyll, which prohibits the growth of bacteria. It also relieves the pain of sore throat.

Cloves

Cloves have potent antibacterial properties that help heal sore throats. It also has anti-inflammatory properties that soothe the swelling and pain.

Goldenseal

This is a potent herbal germ-buster. It can kill bacteria and viruses and at the same time soothe the inflammation in the throat.

Echinacea

This herb is a potent virus-killer. It also boosts the body's immune system to help fight infections.

Sage

This leafy herb is known for its antibacterial properties that can treat sore throat.

Apple Cider Gargle

Ingredients:

- 1 tablespoon apple cider vinegar

- 1 teaspoon salt

- 1 glass of warm water

Procedure:

- Combine everything.

- Use as gargle several times in a day as needed.

OR (milder mix)

Ingredients:

- ¼ cup of apple cider vinegar

- ¼ cup honey

Procedure:

- Mix the 2 ingredients and store in a closed jar.

- Drink 1 tablespoon every 4 hours, as needed until symptoms disappear.

Honey, Lemon and Ginger Gargle

Ingredients:

- 1 teaspoon powdered ginger

- 1 teaspoon honey

- ½ cup hot water

- Juice of half a lemon

Procedure:

- Place the powdered ginger in a cup. Pour the hot water.

- Add lemon and honey.

- Gargle as needed.

Herbal Sore Throat Gargle

Ingredients:

- 1 tablespoon organic sage leaves (fresh or dried)

- 1 cup boiling water

- 1 teaspoon apple cider vinegar

- 1 teaspoon raw honey

Instructions:

- Steep the sage leaves in a cup of boiling water for 10 minutes.

- Strain and place in a separate container.

- Add the apple cider vinegar and honey.

- Gargle at least 4 times a day.

- Continue using until the symptoms of sore throat are relieved.

Chapter 3 Natural Antibiotic Recipes for Cough

Cough is a symptom related to an infection within the respiratory system. It can be of bacterial or viral origins. Chemical cough remedies often have negative side effects, especially if taken for a long period. There are several foods that can help combat these infections in order to relieve cough.

Foods that relieve cough

Garlic

Garlic is often used for cough symptoms related to cold and flu infections.

Lemon

This fruit is best known for its abundant vitamin C content. This vitamin boosts the immune system and makes it stronger against bacterial and viral invasion. Lemon also promotes an acidic environment, which is inhospitable to bacteria and most viruses.

Turmeric

The compound cucurmin has very powerful antibacterial and antiviral properties that help clear up infections that cause cough symptoms.

Cinnamon

This spice has potent antibacterial properties. It is also very effective in relieving cough symptoms.

Echinacea

This herb is also effective in fighting infections that cause cough symptoms.

Apple Cider Vinegar

This is known to be a potent anti-infective agent. It can effectively kill bacteria and viruses by creating a hostile acidic setting within the body.

Sage

This leafy herb has great antibacterial and antiviral properties that help relieve cough, as well as sore throat and fever.

Other herbs for cough:

The following herbs have antiviral properties that relieve cough symptoms:

- Astragalus

- Hyssop

- Lemon balm

- Lemon thyme

- Lemongrass

- Ginger root

Homemade Natural Cough Syrup

Ingredients:

- 1 tablespoon apple cider vinegar

- 1 tablespoon Manuka honey

Procedure:

- Mix the 2 ingredients together.

- Take 2 to 3 times a day, as needed, until the cough disappears.

Antiviral Cough Syrup

Ingredients:

- 1 tablespoon astralagus

- 1 tablespoon lemon balm

- 1 tablespoon lemongrass

- 1 tablespoon hyssop

- 1 tablespoon lemon thyme

- 1 teaspoon of freshly grated ginger

- 1 quart water

- 1 pint raw honey

- ¼ cup vegetable glycerin

Procedure:

- Bring the water to a boil in a small saucepan over medium heat.

- Turn the heat down.

- Add the herbs and cover.

- Let the herbs steep in the water for 30 minutes.

- Strain and remove the herbs.

- Return the liquid to the saucepan and simmer until the liquid is reduced to 1 pint.

- Add the honey and vegetable glycerin.

- Cool.

- Place in a bottle and cover tightly.

- Take 1 teaspoon for a child or 1 tablespoon for an adult, every 4 hours until cough symptoms disappear.

- This cough syrup keeps up to 2 months when in the refrigerator.

Thyme & Manuka Honey Tea Cough Treatment

Thyme helps in expectorating the mucus while the Manuka honey kills bacteria that causes cough.

Ingredients:

- 2 tablespoons fresh thyme (or 1 teaspoon if using dried thyme)

- 1 cup boiling water

- 1 tablespoon of Manuka Honey

- 1 tablespoon freshly squeezed lemon juice

- 1 teaspoon cayenne pepper

- 1 teaspoon turmeric

- 1 teaspoon grated ginger

Procedure:

- Steep fresh thyme in boiling water for at least 10 minutes.

- Add honey, lemon juice and the spices.

- Drink 3 to 4 times a day

Apple Cider and Spice Cough Relief

Ingredients:

- ¼ teaspoon cayenne

- 1 garlic clove, crushed

- ¼ teaspoon raw ginger

- 1 tablespoon apple cider vinegar, organic variety

- 1 tablespoon organic raw honey

Procedure:

- Mix apple cider vinegar, ginger and cayenne.

- Add garlic and honey.

- Shake well.

- Take 1 tablespoon of the mixture as needed until cough resolves or until feeling better.

- Note: the mixture can keep up to 6 months in the refrigerator if stored without the garlic. If garlic is added, the mixture can keep for a week only.

Cough Relief Tea

Ingredients:

- 2 tablespoons chopped fresh sage (or 1 teaspoon if using dried),

- 2 cups of water

- 1 tablespoon raw honey

- 2 tablespoons lemon juice

Procedure:

- Bring the water to a boil. Remove from heat.

- Add the sage leaves.

- Let the leaves steep for 15 minutes.

- Strain the tea.

- Add honey and lemon juice.

- Stir before drinking.

(Mildly) Spicy Cough Relief

Ingredients:

- 3 garlic cloves, chopped

- 3 tablespoons of lemon juice

- 4 tablespoons of raw honey

- ¼ teaspoon of cayenne

- ¼ teaspoon of turmeric

Procedure:

- Mix everything together.

- Take 4 to 5 times daily, as needed when cough symptoms appear.

Chapter 4 Natural Anti-Viral Recipes for Cold & Flu

Flu and colds are viral infections that often recur several times in a year. Pharmaceutical antivirals are very strong. They can cut down sick days by as much as half, but tend to stay long in the body and cause negative side effects.

There is another way to cure viral infections that cause colds and flu. Nature has a lot of foods that can naturally treat these infections.

Foods that treat colds and flu

Ginger

This root has potent antibacterial and antiviral properties that can treat colds and flu in no time.

Garlic

This is a potent anti-infective food. The compound allicin kills off bacteria and creates an inhospitable environment for viruses. A study in 2001 has found that people who ate garlic regularly or took allicin supplements reduced their risk of catching colds by half.

Garlic also contains ajoene, a compound derived from allicin. This compound kills bacteria and inhibits viral reproduction and growth.

Mushrooms

Studies have found that mushrooms have potent anti-tumor, antibacterial and antiviral effects.

Lemon

This citrus fruit is rich in vitamin C and has antibacterial and antiviral properties. It is known to effectively reduce the risk of getting flu and colds. It also reduces sick days when taken regularly.

Sage

This herb has potent antibacterial and antiviral properties that can help fight off colds.

Anise seeds

The seeds have a licorice flavor and have powerful antibacterial properties. It helps to relieve coughs and congestion from colds. Take as tea to treat colds.

Anise Tea for Cold Relief

Ingredients:

- 1 cup anise seeds

- 1 cup hot water

- Pinch of cinnamon

- 1 teaspoon raw or Manuka honey

Procedure:

- Add anise seeds in hot water.

- Steep for a few minutes.

- Add cinnamon and honey.

- Sip.

- Take the tea 3 times daily until cold symptoms are relieved.

Turmeric Tea for Colds

Ingredients:

- ½ teaspoon turmeric powder

- 1 tea bag of mint tea (or 1 teaspoon of loose mint tea)

- ½ teaspoon freshly grated ginger

- 1 teaspoon of fresh mint leaves

- 1 teaspoon lemon juice (or squeeze the juice from half of a lemon)

- 1 teaspoon raw or Manuka honey

Procedure:

- Bring the water to a boil. Remove from heat.

- Steep the mint tea bag in the hot water for 2 to 4 minutes. Or, if using loose mint tea, roll the loose mint tea into a ball and steep in the hot water.

- Add the lemon juice, turmeric and freshly grated ginger. Stir.

- Add honey and mint leaves.

- Strain before drinking.

Cold and Flu-Busting Green Smoothie

Ingredients:

- 1 celery stalk

- 1 peeled lemon

- ¼ of a cucumber

- 1 handful cilantro

- 1 handful parsley

- 1 small ginger root

- 1-2 cups water

Procedure:

- Mix everything in a blender.

- Pulse until smooth.

Cold & Flu Vegetable Juice Remedy

Ingredients:

- 1 celery stalk

- 1 handful parsley

- ½ of a fennel bulb

- 1 turmeric root, the size of a thumb print

- 1 small ginger root, the size of a thumb print

- ½ cup shredded green or purple cabbage

- ½ of a medium-sized green apple

Procedure:

- Mix everything in a blender and pulse until smooth.

Homemade Cold & Flu Infusion

Ingredients:

- 1 lemon

- 1 medium-sized fresh ginger

- Raw honey

Procedure:

- Take the lemon and slice it into quarters.

- Place the lemons in a jar.

- Grate the ginger.

- Add the ginger into the jar of lemons. Stir.

- Add enough honey to cover the lemon and continue stirring.

- Take a tablespoon 3 times per day until symptoms resolve.

Flu and Cold Busting Blend

Ingredients:

- 1 clove garlic, crushed

- ½ cup lemon juice

- 2 tablespoons Manuka honey

- ½ teaspoon cayenne pepper

- 2 tablespoons ginger, grated

- ½ teaspoon cinnamon

Procedure:

- Mix everything in a cup.

- Take 3-4 times a day when feeling under the weather or when suffering from flu.

- Makes several batches to last the day, as this recipe yields only ½ cup, good for 1 dose.

- This blend can be made in large batches and can keep up to 2 days in the refrigerator. Add garlic only when about to drink, and not while in storage.

Raw Mushroom Soup for Colds

Ingredients:

- 8 ounces of mushrooms

- 2 cloves of garlic

- 6-8 ounce of almond milk

- ½ teaspoon salt

- 1 teaspoon peppercorn

- 1 sprig of thyme

Procedure:

- Wash the mushrooms and dry (or drain) them with the caps down.

- Place the mushrooms in a blender and process.

- Pour the almond milk into the blender.

- Add the garlic, salt and peppercorn.

- Blend until a smooth consistency is achieved.

- Stir in the fresh thyme.

- If preferred warm, heat the blended mushroom soup over medium heat for 6 to 8 minutes.

Chapter 5 Antibacterial Foods for Bladder Infections

A wide range of bacterial pathogens causes bladder infections. Most often, this type of infection is recurrent. Taking chemical antibiotics for a long time can cause negative side effects. Bladder infection can be effectively treated with superfoods that have antibacterial properties.

Foods that treat bladder infections

Cranberry

This is probably the most popular antibacterial food used for treating UTIs or urinary tract infections. The flavonols in both cranberry fruit and cranberry juice prevents bacteria from adhering to the walls of the bladder. This will help flush out bacteria better.

Cabbage

Studies have also found cabbage to be effective against urinary tract infections and obstructive-type jaundice.

Cinnamon

This spice has long been used for its medicinal properties. It has very potent antibacterial action, as well as antifungal properties. Studies have shown that cinnamon is effective in fighting UTIs (urinary tract infections) in women.

Garlic and Onions

These contain sulfur compounds that have very powerful antibacterial and antiviral properties that can help in treating bladder infections.

Probiotics (in yogurt)

Probiotics are live beneficial bacteria used for treating several ailments. Recent research has shown that probiotic bacteria are effective at reducing the risk for UTIs. A study has shown that women who took probiotics at least 3 times a week reduced their risk for UTIs by as much as 80%.

Probiotics such a Bifidobacteria and Lactobacilli can be obtained from yogurt, kefir and other fermented foods. It kills bacteria that cause UTI. It also forms a protective barrier around the bladder and vaginal area that can reduce the symptoms of UTI.

Horseradish

This root has been found to be effective at treating recurrent UTIs. The compound AITC (allyl isothiocyanate) can destroy a wide range of bacteria, including *E. coli*. This bacterium is one of the most common bacteria that cause UTI.

Vitamin C

This can be obtained from citrus fruits and some vegetables. Vitamin C promotes acidity in the urinary tract, which inhibits bacterial and viral growth and reproduction. Get vitamin C from the following foods: pomegranate, guava, orange, grapefruit, lime and lemon

Pineapple

The compound bromelain has both antimicrobial and anti-inflammatory effects that help in treating urinary tract infections. Bromelain has been found to fight off bacteria that cause UTI, though experts are not sure exactly how.

Blueberries

Thee small berries are packed with healthy compounds. It has proanthocyanins that prevents *E. coli* from adhering to the cells in the urinary tract. *E. coli* is one of the common bacteria that can cause UTI.

Cabbage with Carrot and Jicama

Ingredients:

- 1 small head of green cabbage, shredded

- 5–6 pieces of medium-sized carrots, grated

- 1 medium-sized jicama, peeled and cut into 1/8" thick sticks

- ¼ cup mint or cilantro leaves, roughly chopped

- ½ red bell pepper, seed removed and sliced into 1/8" thick

- ½ cup freshly squeezed lime juice

- ¼ teaspoon red pepper, crushed

- ¼ cup of maple syrup

- 2 tablespoon of sunflower seeds

- ½ teaspoon salt

Procedure:

- Mix the cilantro (or mint), maple syrup, lime juice, red pepper and salt in a large bowl.

- Add the cabbage, bell peppers, carrots and jicama. Toss to mix everything thoroughly.

- Cover the salad and refrigerate, or serve immediately.

- Garnish with sunflower seeds.

Oriental-Style Cabbage Salad

Ingredients:

- ¼ cup grated purple cabbage

- 1 small head of green cabbage, grated

- 2–3 carrots, grated

- 3 celery stalks, diced

- 1 piece scallion, diced

- 2tablespoon fresh ginger, diced

- 2 cloves of garlic, diced

- 2tablespoon miso

- 2 teaspoons of raw apple cider vinegar

- salt, to taste

- 4 tablespoons of water (or more if needed)

- 1 tablespoon date sugar (or use 2–3 pieces of dates, soaked)

Procedure:

- Mix the vegetables in a large bowl.

- Place the salt, miso, sweetener (date sugar or soaked dates), water and vinegar in a blender. Pulse until smooth and even. Add the ginger and garlic and pulse some more.

- Pour the dressing over the vegetables. Mix well and marinate for an hour while in the refrigerator.

Cranberry Punch with Quince Syrup

Ingredients:

- 2 cups of fresh cranberries

- 6 to 8 medium-sized pears

- 1 cup of quince simple syrup

*For quince syrup

- 3 pieces quinces, medium-sized, slice and remove the seeds

- 1 cup of raw honey

- 2 cups of clean drinking water

Procedure:

- Place the pears and cranberries in a juicer. Juice the fruits.

- Use double strain the juice using a fine mesh strainer in order to remove the cranberry seeds.

- Pour the strained juice in a pitcher. Add the quince syrup. Mix well.

- Put ice in a tall glass and pour the cranberry fruit mix.

*For the quince syrup

- Place the quince, honey and water in a small pot.

- Place over medium heat and bring the mix to a boil.

- Reduce the heat to a simmer.

- Simmer until the fruit turns soft, about 10 minutes.

- Remove the pot from heat.

- Strain and discard the quince. Cool the liquid to room temperature before using.

Cranberry Juice Mix

Ingredients:

- ¼ cup fresh cranberries

- 1 cup fresh blueberries

- 1 small slice of watermelon

Procedure:

- Place everything in a juicer and process.

- Strain the juice and serve.

- Drink 3 times daily until symptoms are relieved.

Conclusion

Thank you again for downloading this book, *"Healing Naturally: 25 Organic Antibiotics and Antivirals Recipes for healing"*.

I hope this book was able to help you find out more about foods that contain potent antibacterial and antiviral properties.

The next step is to throw out all those chemical antibacterial and antiviral drugs. Start eating healthy foods, even if you have no active infections. Living a healthy lifestyle is the best way to avoid illnesses. As they say, an ounce of prevention is better than a pound of cure.

Also, tell everyone about these wonderful foods. Spread the word about the natural ways to combat infections.

Again, thank you.

Enjoy this book?

Please leave a review below and let us know what you liked about this book by clicking on the Amazon image below.

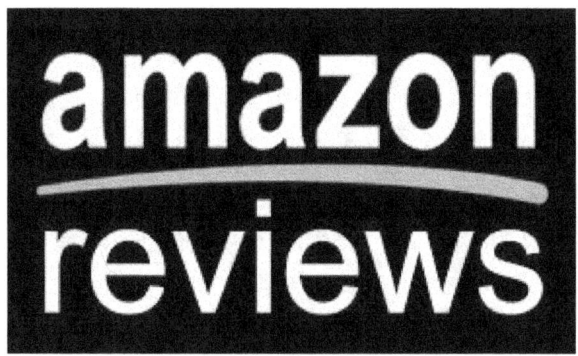

and click on Digital Orders.

The above link directs to Amazon.com. Please change the .com to your own country extension.

www.ingramcontent.com/pod-product-compliance
Lightning Source LLC
Chambersburg PA
CBHW081758280526
45789CB00008B/2911